Dual Control or Certain Derailment

Dual Control

or

Certain Derailment

...Speed is a Given

Miroslaw Manicki
MD, MPH
Kenneth Tingey
PhD, Masters of Pacific International Relations, MBA
Larry Farnes
PT
Dejan Ostojić
MSc, DHM
CIMH GLOBAL/2020 PROGRAM FOR GLOBAL HEALTH
http://2020globalhealth.com
ken.tingey@2020globalhealth.com

Dual Control or Certain Derailment
...Speed is a Given

Miroslaw Manicki, Kenneth Tingey,
Larry Farnes and Dejan Ostojić

ISBN-13: 978-1494858841

ISBN-10: 1494858843

Copyright © 2014, CIMH Global

Logan, Utah/Warsaw, Poland

The cover photograph is used under the following license:

This file is licensed under the Creative Commons license.
You are free:
- **to share** – to copy, distribute and transmit the work
- **to remix** – to adapt the work

Under the following conditions:
- **attribution** – You must attribute the work in the manner specified by the author or licensor (but not in any way that suggests that they endorse you or your use of the work).
- **share alike** – If you alter, transform, or build upon this work, you may distribute the resulting work only under the same or similar license to this one.

This licensing tag was added to this file as part of the GFDL licensing update. It can be found at:
http://en.wikipedia.org/wiki/File:JR-Maglev-MLX01-2.jpg.

According to Wikipedia as of December 31, 2013, the JR-Maglev MLX01 magnetic-levitation train is the unconventional world speed record holder at 581 km/h, or 361.0 mph.

Table of Contents

Public policy "off the tracks"..1
Dual control in principle...3
Dual control and legitimacy..5
Once off the rails, statism beckons..7
Dual control and medicine: The Polish experience..9
    1990: Extraction from top-down dominance..9
    1990-1998: Beginnings of a vertical control aspect................................10
    1999-2003: A closer look at resource transfers.......................................11
    2003: Single payer authority while encouraging a horizontal control structure...13
    Epilogue: Reasserting top-down dominance, with a twist.......................14
Dual control on a national level and the lessons of the last century......16
    What worked...16
        Pulling out of the Great Depression in America.................................16
        Multilateralism and tough love..17
    What didn't work..18
        The Soviet experiment with top-down dominance..............................18
        The Hundred Flowers Campaign and the Great Leap Forward............20
Desire for permanent solutions..22
Examples of effective dual control regimes...23
    Open source software development...23
    Musical composition and performance..24
    Sports performance..26
    Certain longstanding markets..27
Expressive knowledge, the breakthrough we need...29
The inflection point that is our time...31
    Murkiness...31
    Clarity..33
    Urgency..34

Public policy "off the tracks"

We live in a time of great promise to be sure, but current conditions conspire against effective policy implementation on national and international levels. Defeat can be seen at every turn; financial disturbances almost always mirror more fundamental fiscal and social limitations. Policies and procedures, carefully drawn up, are routinely ignored. Front line actors function without the benefit of expert guidance, they routinely exercise their option to ignore rules altogether. The reputation of government programs is severely damaged. Precious resources are thus wasted. Legitimacy suffers.

Such failures encourage bad behavior. As a result, corruption has become the norm. Whether dealing with the physical sciences or with the nuances of sociality and personal preference, no one dares take on the complexities of reality. The expectation that systems will substantially under-perform has become institutionalized.

Thus, no matter how well-intentioned, policy is doomed to break down at some point. Complexity will overpower trite solutions, as nature will never effectively be "gamed". Changing conditions will outpace the policy framework. Systemic weaknesses will eventually be discovered and exploited by those who would corrupt the process. Without a coherent means of staying on track, without a clearly-defined model, the system will eventually exhaust itself, laying itself open to compromise and disintegration.

The problem is not structural; it is not political. There is no credible challenge to the status quo from a political standpoint, nor from the perspective of economics and finance. The problem is that the prevalent governance model is not working. The problem is a procedural one, technical at its core, but with larger implications. Governments and private enterprises alike are crippled by ineffective technologies and systematic disempowerment of knowledgeable, prepared individuals. People exist who know what needs to be done, but they lack viable means of leveraging their knowledge.

If resolution were to come from technologists themselves, it would have occurred decades ago. As the sole source of solutions as they exist, they are rewarded whether systems are effective or not, and they are preconditioned to enjoy the perquisites of power that result from our imbalanced state.

In such an environment, innovators do not even have a framework to understand the problem, let alone find a way out. Think of the issue in this way: If there was a way to capture the best available knowledge, given each situation, and use that knowledge to determine the best outcomes, navigation through even complex journeys could occur with consistency and confidence. Better yet, if such information could be perpetually overseen by specialists who were knowledgeable about each question, armed with the capacity to fix problems that arose, process failure – *derailment* – would be rare indeed.

In this essay, we consider the implications of such a model. The technology in question is available, though not well-known. We refer to the organizational model as "dual control". We describe the phenomenon to some degree, control referring to control of processes in each case, not subjugation of people in any way – very much the contrary. The capability we refer to, systematic empowerment of subject matter experts and authorities to consistently bridge between their knowledge, technologies and models, and the requirements of the rest of us, is referred to as "fluidity". Neither fluidity or detailed elements of the technology in question are considered in any detail herein, but such information is available elsewhere.[1]

---

[1] Tingey, K. B. 2013. *The angels are in the details.* Logan, UT: Profundities LLC/Createspace; Tingey, K. B., Manicki, M. W., and Farnes, L. D. 2013. *2020 Program for Global Health.* Logan, UT/Warsaw, Poland: Createspace/CIMH Global; Tingey, K. B. 2009. *Methods-based management.* San Diego, CA: University Readers, Inc.

Dual control in principle

Dual control is a state of organizational grace where top-down, authoritative control coexists with horizontal, market or social network means of control of processes that support the mission of the organization and its constituents and partners. Achieving dual control is a challenging prospect, as it represents something of a paradox. While authoritative control tends toward absolute, centralized control of resources and authorities, horizontal control mechanisms tend to be distributed among actors that "earn their stripes" by virtue of their expertise and unique capabilities. Their standing results from the judgment of many, not always in ways that are obvious to third parties.

There are checks and balances between the parties, but proponents of authoritative control tend to have the trump card, the last say as to where horizontal forms of control can even exist in the system or sector. They exert primary control over resources, monetary and otherwise.

This is not to say that horizontal control actors don't have the power to grant or take away an organization's relevance and the popularity of its offerings, but authoritative cooperation if not supported is an existential thing. Authorities can shut down horizontal control networks directly by cutting off their resources or achieve similar objectives through inattention and mismanagement. Furthermore, authorities can destroy horizontal networks purposefully. The motives may be simply from jealousy or misunderstanding. They may wish to exert arbitrary behavior that would be more difficult with "experts" on the scene. As organizational leaders control resources as well as administer public missions, their support is critical, particularly where programs, relationships, and networks are in the formative stages. Continued sponsorship and support of authorities is necessary to keep networks of cooperative parties alive, as such relationships tend to grow from tender shoots.

The horizontal network can also suffer from regime change issues, even a change in political leadership. Indeed, though a major aspect of governance should be the protection and nurturing of the horizontal network regardless of political doctrine. One of the major problems in top-down reform efforts is that much of the good from the perspective of the horizontal network gets "thrown out, like the baby with the bath water". This is to say that in such cases, there are inappropriate linkages between the top-down and the horizontal network structures.

This has been identified as a major problem for countries that formerly suffered from repressive and unbalanced command-and-control structures. Even in such conditions, some programs and priorities were effective, particularly in social areas such as health and medicine. As has been pointed out, paraphrased here, reforms should set reality "on its feet, and not on its head".[2]

This essay outlines the importance of this dual form of rationality in government, health, and human services. The principles apply to all fields, but most particularly to environments where complexity and change conspire to make it difficult to manage.

Though "soft skills" must be encouraged and supported in achieving an ongoing balance between authoritative and expert-driven forms of control, there are specific technological requirements as well, which we consider herein to a degree. We look at relevant historical developments from the perspective of dual control. Furthermore, we address opportunities for improvement from this perspective, also considering the benefits of fluidity and expressive knowledge, both of which are described to a degree.

---

[2] Calhoun, C. J. et al. (Eds.). 2002. *Classical sociological theory.* Hoboken, NJ: Wiley-Blackwell, 20-23.

Dual control and legitimacy

Dual control supports the legitimacy of organizations and sectors in two ways. First, it provides a mechanism to control and manage the resources of the organization, including the basic relationships among employees and partners. This is normally described as vertical control, the fundamental authoritative model that supports the activities of the enterprise. Typical computer systems support the vertical model to a degree, along with fairly faithful support of financial accounting and finance models.

The second form of control, the horizontal control of the unique process in question, demands a different model. Although this form of control is common and is essential in order to achieve consistent, successful outcomes, it is typically poorly supported from a technological standpoint. In some cases, once organizational legitimacy is established, this second form of control, that of community, market, and network, suffers from insufficient support, if not actual hostility and attempts at closure.

There is a natural power struggle along these lines. Constant vigilance is required in order to achieve a workable balance. More often than not, authoritative, institutional dominance exists. As was observed at a large religious educational institution, the school's president acknowledged both the "free will" of the students and his right "to enforce it".

When considering the requirements of horizontal control, we do not make reference to "window dressing", nor to any level of condescension. In a state of dual control, authoritative parties do not receive consultation from the membership of the horizontal network; there isn't even oversight other than from the parameters of financial, budgetary matters and legal imperatives, which themselves need to be intricately woven into the functionality of the supporting systems. In a dual control environment, horizontal, network, or market-oriented control means control. Based on their standing in the scientific and practice communities in question, and on the trust and respect granted to them by society and the system at large, they are granted full authority to evaluate and act upon the situations presented therein, utilizing both their knowledge and available data and other forms of information.

The point is, in many cases, non-experts wouldn't even begin to understand what the experts were talking about, nor the implications of various options, nor even the many nuances that would make up the problems sets in their entirety. In complex fields, conditions must exist such that such experts and authorities can get deeply enough into their fields that they are not constrained by the lay dialog.

Authoritative parties would need to have a say with regard to questions of money and the commitment of resources. In an environment of fluidity, such factors could be embedded within the system, the details having been worked out in the abstract. As a result, actions could be carried out and outcomes could be carried out with a minimum of cost, according to the best available knowledge, with immediate access to outcomes data.

Once off the rails, statism beckons

Is there too much top-down authority? The system veers off the rails, the result of a lack of validity. Decisions requiring expert knowledge are made due to political or social factors. Is there too little top-down authority? Chaos results, as the horizontal network lacks the support it needs to survive. Well-meaning individuals and organizations, with the knowledge of what needs to be done, lack the resources to carry out such steps. Perhaps they can help their close circle of friends and their loved ones, but the scope of their influence is limited. In this, they will likely face resistance or legal sanctions from top-down directives that work against nature.

Faced with repression or chaos, history has shown that people end up with the former. This may not be due to choice, as chaos serves as a backdrop for tyrants and thugs. Witness the rise of the Nazi regime, even the environment in Russia after the death of Lenin. Multilateralism was created for this very purpose. The point is to provide scaffolding for a broad political base that allows for such choices to be made by the people as a whole.

The dual control issue has not gone without commentary in this regard. Conversion from "command-and-control" to "market-based" economies requires a "friendly environment", where "top-down control of the resources and processes" are "complemented by horizontal control of the processes of the network". These are called "home-grown policies" introduced by "civil society".

The typical discourse does not expound on fluidity or mastery of communications mediums and networks by experts and authorities. This is critical to success. What may be called home-grown can mask high levels of expertise, as well as essential knowledge of society and culture.

It has been noted that failed "home-grown policies" have typically been thus replaced by "statism, one step at a time" when the dual control model falters. Statism is equivalent to nationalism, where the government asserts direct control and oversight of people and organizations, a universally abhorred condition – other than perhaps by some who would enjoy asserting arbitrary power over others.

Failure to establish and maintain a desirable dual control environment can be due to technical limitations, the smothering effect of top down imperatives, or insufficient support over time. Encroaching statism results in the rise of "neo-command-and-control models", which become poorly regulated and chaotic. In such conditions, a state of prerogative surfaces, though more nuanced than the old command-and-control approach due to the existence of democratic legal frameworks that did not exist before. Ignoring such laws can be awkward at first, but the more everyone pretends that everything is fine, it becomes more and more easy to do whatever you want.

Absent knowledge-based inputs and requisite powers, optimal outcomes simply cannot be achieved. In wholly authoritarian environments, regardless of the professed wishes of the leadership or the people, "information silos" are inevitable. Who is going to collaborate horizontally with peers when it is the pleasing of one's superiors, particular authoritative parties, that determines acceptability and distributes rewards and punishments? Left without effective, timely, guidance from experts in the many aspects of nature that affect well-being and sustainability, modernity, advancement, and general prosperity vanish.

Such conditions affect health systems in particular. Without dual control, health policies degenerate, outcomes worsen, and costs rise to unsustainable levels. Such conditions have resulted in regime failures from all political frames of reference.

Dual control and medicine: The Polish experience

Poland, due to its unique geographical positioning and the high levels of education and accomplishment of its people, has experienced more than its share of reform, revolution, and restitution. In particular, Poland has been a trend-setter in regional and domestic social and economic development. Although in the past, Polish reformers and policymakers did not have access to technologies supporting fluidity and related conceptual models, dual control has been a success factor when the windows of opportunity for health reforms appeared. Failures have occurred when the dual control philosophy has been avoided or postponed. Such relationships are outlined at this point.

1990: Extraction from top-down dominance

Inherited from the previous regime in Poland, top-down control existed with limited horizontal control elements. The system consisted of a homogenous public health care delivery model that had its own control structures, with passive subsidization. This is to say that health providers got paid as long as their work followed plausible patterns. A structurally integrated provider network was paid from a strict line item budget process that could operate more or less effectively under invariable top-down, authoritative control.

With the breakdown of authoritative systems throughout the world at the end of the Cold War, there was a movement toward liberal markets in Poland and elsewhere. Such was a time of great faith in market-related forces. In a sense, markets can be considered as dual control, horizontal control networks, but they do not necessarily incorporate all aspects of dual control as we conceive of it.

Markets, it was hoped in Poland and elsewhere, would behave rationally and fairly, not only supporting a distribution of wealth, but improving the lifestyles of the people. Classical economics was held at the time in high regard, with faith in the famous "invisible hand" that would serve to optimize the enjoyment of customers while rationally distribute the rewards, even in such cases where fairness with regard to income and wealth distribution was out of the question.

Actions taken at that time were rational from a dual control perspective, but there were two problematic areas. First, much too much faith was placed in the beneficial effect of markets as left to themselves. As has been reinforced in worldwide crises since that time, perfect markets, where balance is automatically achieved, are few and far between. This is particularly true of complex, science-based areas such as health and medicine, where conflicts of interest are plentiful and knowledge of various forms are important factors.

Second, technology was not available at that time such that the cognitive aspects of complex problems could be organized and made available to parties involved in the many aspects of health and medicine.[3] Thus, there were many gaps between the science and the practice; prices and quality of services became progressively less rational, varying widely. Not only did many suffer from all socioeconomic classes, resources and programs shot off in directions that were in the best interests of no one. With little or no improvement in terms of outcomes, costs began to skyrocket.

1990-1998: Beginnings of a vertical control aspect

In the early reform period, rapid expansion of the private sector, operating on what was understood as free market principles, committed to a fee-for-service formula. This brought mixed results, not experienced in the prior top-down regime. The safety net, for one thing, largely disappeared. Providers largely directed

---

[3] Actually, there was a seedbed of activity in the American West in this respect, but it was not well-known. Also, it was limited to the large-scale manufacturing sector.

their efforts at what they perceived were promising market opportunities. Personal gain, to be sure, was a motive, but in the absence of a central plan, economic survival was not far from the minds of such individuals and groups.

The question was raised, should there be one system to deal with such outcomes, or should there be two? Was one incentive structure and management philosophy sufficient or should there be two – or more? Ultimately, the choice was made to consolidate activities into one philosophical model. Authority would be represented by a single payer organization, not a government agency, but an independent unit. This new organization was to be answerable to government but free to arbitrate between the needs of the people as represented by the horizontal network of providers and the people themselves. This needed to support authoritative controls and constraints as defined by government.

The object was to establish uniform rules while sponsoring programs to enhance the cohesiveness and scientific rigor of the various groups in health and medical networks. This included providers as well as advocates and the people, allowing them to work through the details of providing services and being responsible for outcomes.

Such a combination of efforts to follow dual control principles was considered to be the only chance to make the operation successful. Our experiences over the years have shown that deviations from this rule have had fatal consequences.

1999-2003: A closer look at resource transfers

Central to the dual control approach employed in that period, the perception was that an improved process was needed to oversee the transfer of resources. Resource transfer took place from the people to government through taxes and other levies. Value was then transferred from government back to the people in the form of services and associated supplies.

A level of rationality was needed on the part of government to carry this out. Governmental involvement in providing such services was justified because of its ability to exert power and authority in the interest of the people in areas that were fundamental, critical to their well-being. In Poland at the time, work went into introduction of the social health insurance model, followed by further development of a payment control mechanism that would do a better job of distributing funds and controlling costs than could be done by the people alone.

As a result of the political consensus reaching process, a unified social health insurance model was devised by the country's sixteen independent regional sickness funds complemented by separate fund for army and police. They agreed to coordinate their activities through the *National Association of Sickness Funds*. This point was to provide a more rational, networked decision process.

Without any obvious political or financial motive, the *Association* was discontinued after two years. At that point, the health program lost much of its horizontal, dual control foundation. In retrospect, it seems that closure of the *Association* occurred as an oversight; there was a lack of awareness of the critical nature of its contribution and a lack of appreciation for the ongoing need for horizontal control mechanisms in Poland's health and medical infrastructure.

Lack of coordination resulted in growing imbalances in contracting models, and finally, in growing inequities in access to health care services in different regions. The health system lost its groundings, lacking the validity and scientific rigor that could be provided only by a strong, vibrant horizontal network, which had provided the foundation of the program. Attempts to merge the regional sickness funds did not fill that gap.

2003: Single payer authority while encouraging a horizontal control structure

The country then established a single payer model that could have supported more effective dual control features, but it suffered from a weakened horizontal model, significantly hampering prospects for success and the validity of system outcomes. To resolve this problem, efforts were taken to support the horizontal "foundation" of the system and to control outcomes in favorable ways. There needed to be a much more organized way of identifying and to fortifying effective procedures within provider networks.

The country's consolidated single payer organization enlisted working groups, including the wide range of stakeholders, into a comprehensive program for defining procedures, areas of coverage, and pricing mechanisms. Self-governance of health and medical communities was an underlying theme, as the unified program worked out detailed plans with dozens of professional working groups and parties representing the hundreds of hospitals in the country.

Services were identified, prices were negotiated, and priorities were established by informed parties, each in their respective areas of expertise. In principle, the matrix of issues and commitments was more complex and nuanced than could be understood by lay people. Ultimately, the validity of such decisions must be grounded in trust, which itself is underscored by interactions within the community.

By all accounts, these conditions were in evidence. This was clearly an initiative to promote collaboration by members of a horizontal, knowledge-based control network. This network was designed to support system uniformity in a repeated fashion. Having achieved order at one level, they would negotiate with the government to apply funds and reinforce initiatives in line with these priorities. From the professional point of view, it was clear that the shift towards the structurally integrated single payer was rational because the individual sickness funds were too small to shoulder growing health care costs, especially when the *Association* was no longer available to manage it.

To avoid unnecessary "dickering" [arguing] over economic issues, the negotiators made use of a "point" system that would later be assigned a monetary value. This was a useful and important feature of the program, allowing participants to concentrate on issues of scientific and practical merit.

In addition to the broad community of participants, the program introduced a consistent, annual review process that dovetailed with the cycles of the top-down, authoritative model used by the government's health ministry. Whereas the ministry represented government's priorities and pronouncements, the payer organization represented the interest of the people as negotiated with the community of scientific and provider groups.

Although a detailed, systematic dual control model was not available, certainly not as made possible by the existence of a fluid technological environment, the combination of activities between the Polish health ministry, the authorized payment channel, and the many provider groups, resulted in successful outcomes. The enlistment of the many experts and authorities within the working groups brought substantially improved outcomes and other mutual goals.

Epilogue: Reasserting top-down dominance, with a twist

Lamentably, gains from having built the horizontal, science and medical network were fleeting. Turnover, particularly at the government level, brought in individuals and programs that were not well-informed, nor committed to carry out needed actions to refine and support the horizontal network.

The annual service planning process that had shown to be so effective was the first such function to break down. Within a few budgetary cycles, without the flow of information and the opportunity for mutual commitment for ongoing consultation, the effectiveness of the horizontal network and its interactions with the authoritative control structure melted away.

In the place of the professional, scientific network of services and control, the government appointed staff members with medical and scientific credentials, to be sure, but without direct authority, nor understanding and commitment to the dual control model that had been painstakingly established.

The idea was that such individuals were to provide advice and guidance equivalent to those of participants in the horizontal network. In reality, they did little to support the legitimacy of that network. From their positions within the top-down, authoritative structure, they served to undermine the horizontal network, upsetting what balance existed in the wake of the program's unraveling from other forces. Eventually, even indirect connections with scientific and practice communities broke down as the administration's experts were released or moved on to other activities.

As a result, policies were deployed with little or no consultation, let alone collaboration. In complex and changing areas such as health and medicine, top-down mandates alone have not been shown to match the requirements of nature and the needs of the people. Much of this occurred under the rubric of "regulation," but resulting policies and systems surfaced with little to do with nature's regulatory processes, which are not subject to negotiation. Such one-sided, uninformed policy frameworks resulted in severe resistance from powerful stakeholders in the country's health and medical sectors, particularly the medical chamber, the nursing chamber, and professional associations and trade unions. Furthermore, budgets grew uncontrollably and many social and health-related ills have persisted, if not having deteriorated during this period.

Dual control on a national level and the lessons of the last century

Although we are considering the technological and methodical aspects of dual control, which are new to the policy dialog, dual control concepts are not new to public affairs. On the contrary, they are central to issues of government legitimacy and social stability. This is substantiated by many developments, a few of which are outlined herein.

What worked

Pulling out of the Great Depression in America

As described in Poland in the 1990s, market forces alone did not bring desired outcomes. Specific and concrete plans needed to be put into effect that lined up authoritative as well as expertise or market-related controls. Such was also the case in the United States decades earlier with efforts to stimulate the economy in the face of economic depression and social stagnancy. As described at the time by Marriner Eccles, a commercial banker who later assumed policy positions in the U. S. Treasury and the Federal Reserve, programs needed to be put into effect that would put money into the hands of many, providing them with the ability to purchase goods and services. In this way, they would serve to stimulate the economy, reversing the downward trends in effect at that time.

Policy makers insisted on local controls in the dissemination and management of such funds and related programs. As Eccles himself indicated, decisions and programs needed to be organized at the local level, where people were informed and knowledgeable about local conditions. Particular efforts were taken to sponsor programs in engineering, construction, natural resources, and transportation as well as in the arts, in music, painting, sculpture, etc. Programs were overseen by the communities themselves.

This resulted in innovations and outcomes that have survived the test of time.

Multilateralism and tough love

As an extension of works programs successes in the United States and in line with desires for rectifying disastrous results from the Treaty of Versailles from World War I, international development programs were established after World War II that demonstrated important dual control elements. These programs were established based on the principals of U. S. works programs as described above. Thus, they were careful to integrate technical and social elements with investment decisions and other programs.

Resulting from this was the World Bank and many additional development organizations based on these philosophies, including those sponsored by the United Nations, the European Commission, and other national and other regional development organizations. These efforts resulted in a proud tradition in economic development, the establishment of prosperity and peace throughout the world. The model in question, financial control as established in an hierarchical manner coupled with expertise, much of it local, has brought infrastructure to many countries of the world and has developed ongoing capacity in most cases.

One challenge faced by these programs is brought on by the need to sponsor horizontal networks in far-flung nations, many of them in their nascent stages in terms of democracy and legal protections. In many cases, funds are expropriated from projects by locals. To the extent that funds and other resources are thus contravened, the projects can become counterproductive, encouraging oppressive, top-down regimes or just corruption in general. In such cases, horizontal control could better be achieved through the use of technologies that support more detailed processes. On the other hand, the promise of support for local development can be used to support sustainable, democratic innovations in-country.

What didn't work

The Soviet experiment with top-down dominance

In the aftermath of the revolution of 1919, Bolshevik leaders faced a stark reality. The economy of Russia was not the advanced, multifaceted collection of industries as existed in Great Britain or Germany. Mostly agrarian, the economy of Russia left much to be desired from a modernist perspective. Lenin started out as a pragmatist, enlisting the efforts of entrepreneurs, the American Armand Hammer being the most famous of these. This was Lenin's "New Economic Policy", the NEP. The point was to reward entrepreneurs for establishing new industrial capacity. Monopolies in needed sectors were offered to such individuals. These amounted to horizontal networks, where control and commerce served to grow the Russian economy. Mr. Hammer got several concessions of this kind, including markets for tractors (he sold Fords), pens, and pencils. He represented thirty-seven American companies in all, selling products to Russia through the NEP until local manufacture could be arranged. For the pencils, he imported an entire town from Germany that knew the technology and the trade. This was horizontal control, indeed.

Stalin had a different view. His vertical authoritative system shut down the NEP, the horizontal one. Fortunately Mr. Hammer suffered a less severe fate than many Russians at the behest of Mr. Stalin. He was paid off in Faberge eggs and other jewels of the realm, which he proceeded to sell from a shop he set up in the Empire State Building in New York City.

After Lenin's death, Stalin started out in a defensible way to craft an economic program. He pitted two Russian economists against each other, Bukharin and Preobrazhensky, in a famous public debate. Bukharin was a proponent of what we may call dual control, a balance of authoritative and market, or expert-driven, factors. This focused on innovations by small businesses, farmers, and the like. Preobrazhensky argued for a top-down model exclusively, based on heavy industry, state-run, large-scale industries and little or no input from private interests or agricultural producers.

Once the chips were on the table, Stalin eliminated both contenders from the public arena and then took a position in favor of an authoritarian system more overwhelming in consequence than Preobrazhensky had considered. Coupled with this was a clampdown on any contending sources of income that might distract from his plan for a state-run economy based principally on heavy industry. These actions often turned violent, as was the case in the Ukraine. That was not a time and a place to argue for dual control.

Actually, there is a story about that. After Stalin's death, in a late night meeting in which Nikita Khrushchev was reciting mistakes and atrocities of the prior regime, a voice from the audience called out (we paraphrase) "If he was so bad, why didn't you stop him?" Khrushchev responded forcefully, "Who said that?" When there was no response, he said, "Now you know why."

That did work, for a time, in a way. It did built up the capacity of the nation if not the society of its people. This was an important factor in countering the brutal force of the Nazi regime. But it was not sustainable. It was not fair. This was brought out in the famous "X" essay of George Kennan in 1947. Published in *Foreign Affairs* as being written by the mysterious X, as it wasn't politically acceptable for an essay to be published in such a manner that had been written by an actively-serving government official. It had been sent from the American Embassy in Moscow via cable in three pieces due to its length. Interestingly, a major aspect of the X article was to explain why Russia was not going to participate in the World Bank and the other multilateral initiatives.

It wasn't that the Russian people wouldn't put up with the aggressive top-down model of control, but that they *couldn't*. Kennan's point was that the level of oppression was so overwhelming that the Russian people would eventually throw it off from the force of an existential need. Decades later, this proved correct. It is interesting that the X article was published at all, as it represented a breach of top-down controls within the U.S. government in the view of some.

The Hundred Flowers Campaign and the Great Leap Forward

Mao Zedong's cartoonish notoriety in the West is misplaced. Imperfect though he was, he overcame great odds to unify and put his country on a strong footing. He and Deng Xiaoping in particular have much to offer in understanding this critical factor, in achieving a balance in dual control. Their successes and their failures, particularly their scale, given China's size, resonate in our time.

After the original successes in organizing the Chinese government with the assistance of the Russians, Mao was concerned about the upper class of autocrats that was forming, comprised of politicians, scientists, and technicians. He was also concerned about growing dependence on Russia, which had served to educate and train the Chinese elite. He wished to stimulate a massive round of populism within China to counter the power of a new, controlling elite with a horizontal movement, where ideas would be shared and acted on. He called on an active, healthy dialog stimulate by and emanating from the people. He called this initiative the "hundred flowers" movement, where "a hundred flowers [would] bloom and a hundred schools of thought [would] contend". He didn't really like the ensuing result, so he subsequently called a halt to the process. It was soon followed with his call for a "Great Leap Forward (GLF)", with similar objectives, but with less of a call for input from the masses.

This is standard dual control material. One problem, though, was that the horizontal network to be organized, with all of the "blooming" and "contending", was governed and artificial. In the GLF, some populist ideas for home-based industrialization were introduced, some by Mao and other federalists. Curiously, though

Mao made it obvious that he wanted input, he was far too pushy about the entire process, dictating both process and solution – as in the famous backyard iron forges. For one thing, available experts were among the class of people he was trying to put down. His objective was to disenfranchise, not enable such people. There really wasn't interest in meritorious ideas from other sources.

The net result was catastrophic, resulting in tens of millions of deaths and great social and political unrest. Sponsorship of the horizontal network by authorities is of critical importance. It must be real. There must be a transfer of power based on knowledge and expertise along with a mechanism to continue that process. In the Chinese case, once the imbalance started, it spiraled downward further, contributing to the Cultural Revolution, which turned the country upside down. In that case, experts were purposefully humiliated and dis-empowered, many maimed and killed.

The Chinese tradition provides much material to understand the requirements of dual control from this experience and their response to it. The writings of Deng Xiaoping from the late 1970s are particularly illustrative of their kinds of solutions. His famous "seeking truth from facts" is clearly directed at dual control objectives. The outside world sees China as being obsessed with top down control and this may be true. They do, however have a tradition of sponsorship of horizontal, expert and market-driven control networks, with many successes as well as failures.

Desire for permanent solutions

The point is in the establishment of a policy framework that is consistent and self-sustaining. This is one benefit from an effective horizontal network. Populated and controlled by knowledgeable people and people networked into markets and social networks, horizontal control networks are effective means of preparing for and adapting to the future. With time, commitment, and continued sponsorship, the promise of fluidity is that answers can present themselves with increasing specificity, more clarity, and simplicity. With each iteration, the content can be improved, the solutions can be enhanced, and the general body of knowledge can be expanded upon.

This is the famous goal of policy-makers everywhere, the equivalent to "wishing for more wishes" from Aladdin's genie. We wish to have a self-perpetuating system that can handle change, that can adapt itself, and that can stop hitting up against and start cooperating with nature.

It was the search for a model of permanence, an attempt at dual control, that got Maoist China in trouble in the "Hundred Flowers" initiative and the "Great Leap Forward". This was clearly an attempt to create a horizontal network of experts, not unlike the New Economic Policy in Russia and the efforts in Poland and elsewhere to establish a self-sustaining private sector. Similarly, in the United States during the Great Depression and in the establishment of the World Bank and other multilateral institutions, the object is to sponsor prosperity through openness and continual peace.

Examples of effective dual control regimes

When considering such lofty objectives on the scale of individual nations, it is helpful to see where dual control has been effective and has stood the test of time. Dual control has existed in some form in all human endeavors. Authority and expertise are important bedfellows; one cannot get very far without the other. Of course, there isn't an organization, nor a leader that does not call attention to the need for expertise in the carrying out of their respective missions. This is the case even in organizations where expertise and collaboration is quite severely repressed.

Open source software development

The open source software development community is an interesting phenomenon, one whose existence is a testament to the potential for collaboration by parties with a common interest. The open source movement is the reaction by large organizations with software development capacity to overcome poor support and responsiveness to their needs by commercial providers of software in particular.

It is one thing for technology companies to be less that responsive to typical customers and less than forthcoming about what might be done for them. It is something else to behave in such a manner when customers have extensive technical resources and talent to call upon. In this, we refer to large corporations, government agencies, universities and research institutions, and other big users of computing technologies.

Unhappy with what they were getting from software vendors, many such organizations joined forces beginning in the 1980s to sponsor the development of world class software in an open environment. This meant that they agreed to share and to collaborate. Mutual use of the underlying source code that defined what the software was designed to do has allowed such organizations to leverage the knowledge of their people on a large scale. Resulting products are in many cases superior to their commercial counterparts.

The collaborative efforts provided a fertile environment for developing software of all kinds. Some of the best software came from organizations that were designed specifically for open source efforts. Apache is an example of a very effective program of this kind. Based on its successful web server software, which continues to support roughly half of the 716 million web sites on the Internet, the Apache organization has brought many enterprise-scale projects into use that make use of its well-established methods and procedures.

The open source community is a horizontal network principally sponsored by organizations that made the collective decision to collaborate in an area other than their principal missions, but that was critical to success. This collaboration has proven effective for decades, demonstrating a level of balance that is admirable. Similar projects have resulted in the development of famous, widely-used technologies including the Linux operating system, Mozilla, Eclipse, GIMP, MySQL, Open Office, and many others.

Of course, the open source phenomenon is greatly aided by the fact that participants are capable computer programmers. This is to say that they have and use common languages. This is the point of the exercise. For this reason, the open source movement is an important model with regard to dual control, not only an example of its potential, but a laboratory with lessons to learn in how to carry out dual control in the long term.

Musical composition and performance

Dual control clearly exists in the world of music. The composer is the ultimate arbiter of what was to be done. He or she can lay out musical notes in ways that integrate the work of all ensemble members. As the Italian language is the "lingua franca" of that system, the term "tutti", everyone or everything in that language, came to represent the phenomenon of all performers working together for the good of the whole.

We have pointed this out often as referenced earlier, but the music performance model is such an invaluable example of dual control that this review would not be complete without mention of how it works and its intrinsic benefits.

Here are the basics. Based on a notational system developed over the centuries that has been validated in modern times for its accuracy, the musical model allows highly-skilled composers to design sound-scapes with virtually unlimited creativity. The product of such efforts is a range of compositions that identify and reinforce all aspects of life, all emotions, all human situations. Even natural phenomena are identified, mimicked, and enhanced.

The solution is permanent. The same model used by Beethoven and his contemporaries is used today. Among other things, this means that their works can be performed today. When musicians come together, they have the option of performing the great works at least to the extent of their abilities. Nonetheless, the availability of the great works of music serves to raise performance levels of all musicians. With appropriate guidance and instruction, many can rise to that level, to the benefit of us all.

The innovators that developed the system did so in many small increments. The science of sound was a critical factor. Modern instrumentation provided validation of the correctness of their understanding of sound's characteristics and structures. Technologies had to be developed to allow application of the notation system to all instrument types and to the voice. This took centuries to accomplish. In many cases, generations had to die off for needed innovations to work their way into general usage.

Composers can let their minds soar in the creation of their works. The need to understand the rules, the patterns of melody, harmony, and rhythm that support sound's features as they interpret them. This is referred to as music theory. Such knowledge corresponds with what we refer to herein as "expressive knowledge". Key to the process is the directness and accessibility of the model. Beethoven and his fellow composers, then and now, never had to deal with a management information system (MIS) departments, nor did their music ever need to be approved by anything other than the "court of public opinion". Well, Mozart and some others did have issues with their sponsors at times, but that was a political and artistic issue, not technical.

The result for musicians is a system characterized by high degrees of satisfaction and motivation, also an environment where control is evident. Once the music is laid out and a conductor is in place, top down control is undeniable – particularly in the case of a leader with a strong personality. The performance skills of the instrumentalists and singers, benefiting from a common language, but very different performance requirements, talents, and skills in each case, demonstrate horizontal control at its best. The result, with competent ensembles is a high degree of variety, breathtaking breadth and flexibility, indeed, perfection.

These lessons, we believe, can be transferred and mastered in other organizational contexts, including those of organizations, governments, and other public and private associations.

Sports performance

"That is why they play the game" is a common quotation when it comes to organized sports, whether professional or not. Much can be said about the economics of sports, of movements by management, and by controlling elements, including even the influence and power of coaches, but in the final analysis, it is how the athletes themselves perform in some form of competition that matters, given rules that have been established.

There are payrolls, management declarations, player trades, facilities management issues, uniforms, public relations campaigns, and on and on. The point is that when the buzzer sounds and the game begins, it is the interactions among the players that matter. There is a coach to be sure that may or may not loosen the reigns enough to allow the players to decide the plays to run, but in the final analysis, it is up to the players on the field to perform. Horizontal control of processes takes over when it matters; that is the only thing that counts.

Certain longstanding markets

Some markets come and go, while others persist. The market for corn, for example, the agricultural product, mirrors that of the ascent of man, and most likely stems from earlier struggles among the beasts.

How does such a market exist and persist? How are the various parties in such environments enticed and rewarded? An ongoing dialog exists among the parties in question, with considerations of supply and demand, differentiating the good and the bad, the desirable and the undesirable, and arriving at a level of balance that ultimately survives the test of time. If such conditions do not exist, events overtake perceived imbalances, eventually with longer-term implications. The Corn Laws in England from the 1200s to the mid-nineteenth century are an example of this. Indeed, the founding of the *Economist* magazine was done in part to convince the English government to do away with restrictions on the import of corn and other grains.

How do such persistent, long-term markets endure? Of course, they represent goods and services for which there is ongoing demand, though they must deal with short-term conditions. Gold, for example, is always highly-valued, though its price does fluctuate.

Markets for luxury items depend on such subtleties of communication, resulting in long-term balance in these persistent markets. How are exorbitant prices for jewelry, timepieces, etc., maintained? Someone must know the difference. There must be communication among such parties. There must be ways of validating and verifying. Otherwise, chaos and confusion will result, conditions that scare away buyers, introduce instabilities, and discourage value-based investments.

Such markets must have strong horizontal communication networks where participants enjoy autonomy and trust, and where there ia a means of verifying critical factors. Take the example of the financial markets. These thrive on continuity and trust, but gains are often achieved by means of the opposite. Great gains can be made by predicting shifts before they occur. Hidden wisdom is one factor, as is an ability to identify outliers, the weak and vulnerable, and destroy their credibility.

If there were no rules in such matters, the markets would decay and fall apart. The example of the investor Bill Ackerman and his attack within the equity market on Herbalife, the American herbal products company. As it stands, the company and its supporters have withstood his attacks and the company's price has prevailed, to Mr. Ackerman's embarrassment and loss. If there were no "horizontal" rules of the market, if they did not hold sway in a consistent, dependable manner, capricious attacks within the ranks could succeed based on power and influence alone.

Expressive knowledge, the breakthrough we need

In the face of this, given the ravages of complexity and change, dual control regimes are typically doomed. Surely, authoritarian parties can pass the baton to potential horizontal control communities, but how do such networks function? How do participants manage context and track complexities that exist? This is a challenge even in simpler practice areas, let alone in complex areas such as medicine, human services, economic development, environmental management and the many other complex and changing environments.

Even if models are developed to accomplish such objectives at one time, how can they keep up with change. With time, the forces for chaos find their ways into the system, allowing for corruption and diversion of efforts and resources.

Dual control objectives date to ancient times. Keys to how such objectives can be achieved are also of ancient date. An age of reason described by Plato and later Aristotle envisioned an environment in which reason was granted its aliquot of power. The concept has risen and fallen from grace, typically at the choice of ruling parties, some of who exercised restraint, but granted license in very limited ways. The *Age of Reason* resulted in a rise in expectations. Resulting efforts, though promising at times, failed to prevent wild political and economic fluctuations leading to our times.

Order is the bedfellow of reason, while disorder and confusion are associated with chaos and a lack of control. The key to control itself, to dual control in particular, is an ability to model active processes. Aspects of this were documented by Aristotle in particular. Development of a form of this occurred with the original development of computers, but the tools that were developed were more computer-friendly than people-friendly. Fluidity demands that the opposite be the case.

In 1996, Manuel Castells indicated that power in a system was the ability to control the switches within the system. This is true. As to the needs of governments and of their societies, such investitures of power have yet to take place. When empowerment of experts and authorities is knowingly sponsored and supported, the door is opened to dual control.

As outlined in the table below, there are three functional knowledge types. The first two, tacit and explicit forms of knowledge, are well-known and well-understood. In fact, though the functions outlined under expressive knowledge categories, shaded, may seem arcane and perhaps simplistic, they represent powerful means of defining and managing the knowledge of actions and processes, a critical missing link in the achievement of fluidity.

This is the modern equivalent to the Congo River basin of a century ago. We know more about the far planets than we do about the implications of our own knowledge when applied to an active model. Of course, this needs to be corrected.

		Tacit, Explicit, Expressive Model		
		Desired form of knowledge (TEE model)		
		tacit	*explicit*	*expressive*
Existing form of knowledge	*tacit*	give lecture	write document	**design process**
	explicit	read document	review documents	**transfer process from document**
	expressive	**follow process (as in a simulation)**	**create report from process**	**expand from one process to many**

The inflection point that is our time

The next few years are critical to long-term success in the governance of nations and in the peace and prosperity of the world. We have the knowledge. We have the heritage, both of late and throughout history. We have the resources. We have the people, the good people and fabulous societies of the world.

What we need to do is to knit these together into a lasting fabric, a framework for policy and implementation that can overcome both complexity and change. We need to rise out of our murky present, to achieve a new level of clarity, and to address the challenge with a sense of urgency, showing respect for the nature and impact of imminent failure if we fail to act.

Murkiness

Recently, Larry Farnes called on a medical specialist who was an executive with a large insurance company in the United States. Mr. Farnes indicated to the physician that he had a message, one that would, substantially reduce the need for spinal surgeries. He indicated that due to the procedure in question, based on a comprehensive set of measures among among the muscles and joints of the body, most such operations would not be necessary. Benefits to be gained would be both economic and social.

The specialist agreed that such would likely be true. He consented to a followup meeting. He did mentioned that the insurance company paid for hundreds of millions of dollars in spinal surgeries annually. Mr. Farnes interpreted this statement as an expression of interest in saving the money, etc.

This did not seem to be the case. After a few days, he called to set up the subsequent meeting with no response. After several attempts, the specialist finally gave him the bad news: He couldn't find anyone at the firm to "spearhead" the project. Mr. Farnes mentioned that he thought that the physician would be that person. "Oh, no, I couldn't do that", he said.

Is this an example of dual control? Certainly it is an example of control of some kind. It represents a kind of murkiness in health and medicine and in many other sectors. Clearly, the innovation in question was being rejected out-of-hand, without the opportunity to prove its effectiveness or lack thereof. Power was being manifest to be sure, but in this case, it was the power to ignore, to stave off a form of innovation through inaction, the power to quietly work against the public interest.

To the insurance company, the hundreds of millions in procedures being paid for surely constituted something other than an expense. Perhaps there were fees involved or other countervailing arrangements that caused the insurance company to want to spend the money. No matter the health risks, pain, and disease that results from such disorders. No matter the cost to society.

In the absence of a dual control regimen, there are few options for continuing such innovative efforts as long as powerful organizations behave in such a fashion. In a dual control regimen, new methods procedures would flow into the system based on their merit, with underlying arrangements being negotiated in a balanced environment, where decisions can be made considering the best interests of the people based on the best available knowledge. Such decisions, if supported by fluid technologies, could catch critical issues "upstream", when they can do the most good. The best way to prevent corruption of various kinds is to be vigilant, preventing underlying conditions from surfacing in the first place.

This does not mean that there would not be opportunities for personal and organizational gain in such environments, but dual control would change the rules of the game. Under dual control, where expressive knowledge is present, situations present themselves in more coherent forms. Context is thus preserved. New opportunities emerge, more in light of the needs of healthy people.

Why would an organization with conflicts of interest of this kind be granted the opportunity to kill the very innovations that would benefit their clients the most? Perhaps such imbalances are unimportant in some markets for goods and services. They can hardly be justified, however, where the health of the public is in question. Perhaps the specialist in the insurance company would never relent to steps that would eliminate spinal surgeries as a major health threat. More than likely, he shouldn't be given the opportunity to make that decision in the first place.

Clarity

What would it take for innovative knowledge to reach the market in a dual control environment where fluidity existed? Experts would need to agree on the conditions under which certain health-related steps were to be collected. Scientific as well as financial factors would need to be considered and organized in expressive forms. Agreement would need to be reached among all involved parties, empowered by a single payer authority in each case. This authority needs to be aware and supportive of top down mandates while being functionally integrated with horizontal, knowledge-based processes.

In our complex societies, only singular payment authorities are in position to evaluate the whole of relationships among many parties supporting applicable laws and policies under conditions for which they were established.

There would need to be a veritable "symphony" of voices representing all relevant parties and interests. All of this would need to be presented to the people of the world in easily understood, non-obtrusive ways. Obviously, this presupposes use of the Internet and other available networked resources.

Urgency

We think ourselves as living in modern times. Surely, the mistakes of the past should not be repeated now. Considered from the perspective of dual control, however, we can see a future that is decidedly imbalanced. First of all, who has ever heard of such an arcane concept as dual control? Second of all, the enabling model, expressive knowledge, is even less well-known. Without a felicitous marriage of the two, something in stark contrast to policy regimes as they exist today, nations are left to muddle along with indefinite mandates, loose policy frameworks, and economic and social arrangements characterized by prerogative, ineffective execution, and waste.

Without a clear view of the opportunity to use fluidity and expressive knowledge to support critical requirements of dual control, regimes can be seen to veer in the direction of didactic top-down approaches. Without being prepared to envision a future graced by fluidity and dual control, governments could continue to stumble into top down models that ignore opportunities to meet the stated responsibilities of governments and service providers to their people. Without dual control and the flexibility it brings, policy implementation and governance runs the risk of not being able to respond to complexity or change, resulting in veritable derailments and failures that will skew political prospects and increase the likelihood that corruption and authoritarian caprices will prevail in the nations of the world.

Alphabetical Index

Age of Reason..29
agricultural producers...19
Armand Hammer..18
authoritative control..3, 9, 15
Authority..6, 11pp., 23
authority,...15
bad behavior...1
Beethoven..25p.
beneficial effect of markets...10
Bukharin..18
Castells..30
chaos..7, 27, 29
civil society...7
Clarity..22, 31, 33
complex problems...10
complexities...1, 29
complexity...1, 4, 29, 31, 34
Congo River basin...30
control of processes...3, 27
Corn Laws..27
corruption..1, 17, 29, 34
Deng Xiaoping...20p.
derailment..1p.
dickering..14
Dual control.......................1pp., 9pp., 14, 16pp., 29p., 32pp.
economic survival..11
expectation...1
expert knowledge..7
expertise...3, 13, 16p., 21, 23
expressive knowledge..4, 26, 29p., 32, 34
failures...1, 20p., 34
fluidity...2, 4, 6, 9, 22, 29p., 33p.
free market..10
friendly environment...7
George Kennan..19
Great Depression...16, 22
Great Leap Forward...20, 22

home-grown policies	7
horizontal control	3, 5, 7, 9, 12p., 17p., 22, 26p., 29
horizontal model	13
horizontal network	5, 11p., 14p., 20pp., 24
Hundred Flowers Campaign	20
information silos	8
input	19pp.
knowledge-based	8, 13
legitimacy	5, 15p.
Lenin	18
lingua franca	24
Mao Zedong	20
market-based	7
MIS	26
Multilateralism	7, 17
murkiness	31p.
nationalism	8
negotiation	15
neo-command-and-control	8
NEP	18
New Economic Policy	18, 22
off the tracks	1
Personal gain	11
Policies and procedures	1
policy frameworks	15, 34
Preobrazhensky	18p.
private interests	19
Public policy	1
regime failures	8
regulation,	15
single payer	11, 13
staff members	15
stakeholders	13, 15
Stalin	18p.
statism	7p.
system uniformity	13
Tacit, Explicit, Expressive Model	30
top down control	21, 26
top-down	3, 9p., 14p., 17pp., 34
top-down authority	7
top-down control	7, 9

top-down, authoritative control..3, 9
trust..6, 13, 28
tutti...24
uniform rules..11
Urgency...31, 34
wishing for more wishes...22
World Bank...17, 19, 22
X...19p.

www.ingramcontent.com/pod-product-compliance
Lightning Source LLC
Chambersburg PA
CBHW051824170526
45167CB00005B/2146